Editions L.A.

DIGITAL CREATIVE AGENCY

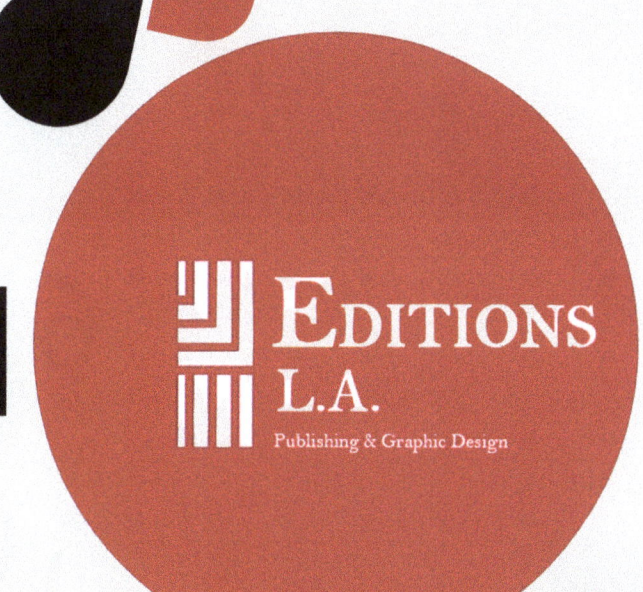

We Transform Your Vision Into Creative Results

Editions L.A. is a full-service agency based in Los Angeles. Our company is a collective of amazing people striving to build delightful services
We believe that is all about getting your message across clearly and with a "Wow!" thrown in for good measure.

Our Awesome Services

Branding

We build, style and tone your brand identity from the ground up.
We rebrand established bands, brands or businesses.

Merchandise Store
Website design and E-Commerce
Website updates

Digital Marketing

CD Cover | Banners | Logo design | Flyers | Brochures | Leaflets | Print ads | Magazine covers & artworks
Facebook / twitter / instagram / youtube artworks
| Book cover
Infographics | Icon Design |
| TshirtsProduct Labels | Presentation slides
Corporate graphics
Professional photo editing & enhancing
Redesign existing elements
YouTube Optimization and Monetization
Youtube Video Editing
Lyric Video and Advertising Design.

Publishing

BOOK COVER DESIGN
EBOOK FORMATTING SERVICES
and distribution on major platforms
(Amazon, Barnes & Nobles..)

Tell us about your dream and we will make it true!

Editions L.A.
7210 Jordan Avenue Suite B42, Canoga Park, California 91303, United States
info@edtions-la.com
Website: www.editions-la.com

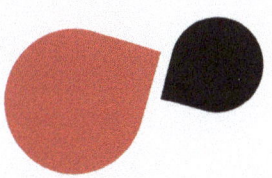

Pump it up Magazine

TABLE OF CONTENTS

⚡ **EDITORIAL**
Page 5

⚡ **MICHAEL B. SUTTON**
C.E.O.
Consultant
Label Owner
Artist & Producer is back with a hot new single
"SEXUAL"

6

⚡ **REVIEW**
Music Frequency
For Your Health

⚡ **WHAT'S HOT**
Eating wel for your mental health
Indie Music Discovery

10

⚡ **FASHION**
Look and Feel Younger
with Black Sed Oil

⚡ **FITNESS**
Get in shape!

18

⚡ **BEAUTY**
How to look expensive

⚡ **Fun Quizz**
Have fun!

27

⚡ **HUMANITARIAN AWARENESS**
Tips for taking care of your mental health
C-PTSD AND NARCISSISTIC ABUSE

Pump it up
MAGAZINE

PUMP IT UP MAGAZINE
LINKS

WEBSITE
www.pumpitupmagazine.com

FACEBOOK
www.facebook.com/pumpitupmagazine

TWITTER
www.twitter.com/pumpitupmag

SOUNDCLOUD
www.soundcloud.com/pumpitupmagazine

INSTAGRAM
pumpitupmagazine

PINTEREST
www.pinterest.com/pumpitupmagazine

PUMP IT UP MAGAZINE
30721 Russell Ranch Road
Suite 140
Westlake Village,
California 91362
United States

📞 (818)514 – 0038(Ext:102)
✉ info@pumpitupmagazine.com

EDITORIAL

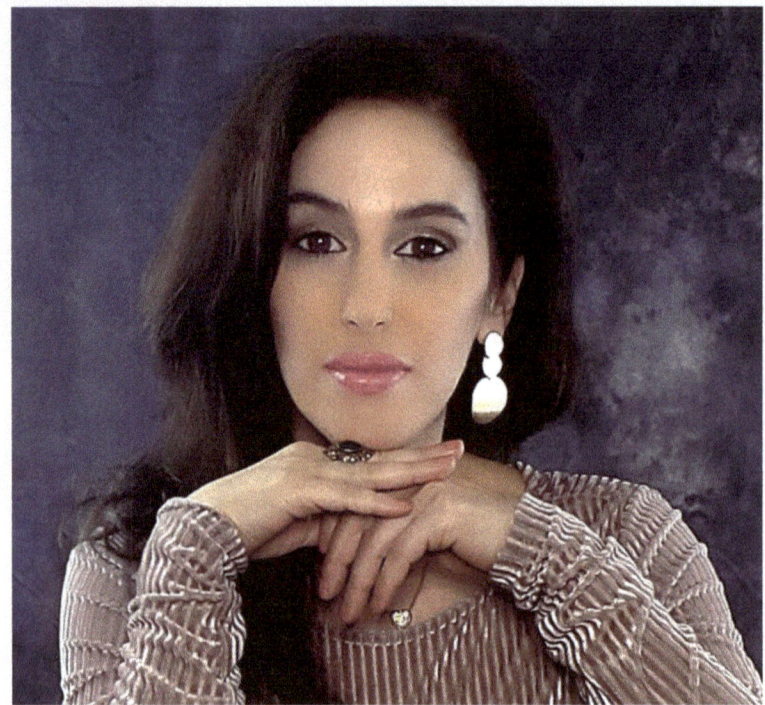

Greetings,

It's time! Pour a cup of tea, grab your favorite magazine, Pump it up Magazine that is!

In this edition, we have a few surprises that we hope will pique your interest and keep you smiling and enjoying Pump It Up Magazine!

We are proud to feature on the cover Michael B. Sutton. An awesome talent and handsome man, inside - out, who has a voice that reminds us of some of the Motown greats! When you hear Stevie Wonder, Marvin Gaye, Smokey Robinson ,Diana Ross, The Temptations, The Jackson Five and The Commodores, you know it's the signatur sound of Motown.

Michael B. Sutton was discovered by Stevie Wonder and has written and or produced songs from Michael and Jermaine Jackson , to Smokey a Robinson and remains active to this day. From the early 60's to the present Motown still is known as the "Sound of Young America" . And there are many other hidden icons from the Motown family.

"Sexual" is the latest in a teasing string of singles leading to the two-decades-awaited release of Michael B. Sutton's as-yet-untitled second album (his first since 2002's Hopeless Romantic.

No doubt Indian Summer shall continue…between the sheets!

Let's Pump up the volume of love, peace, and happiness every day of the year!

Well that's all for now, May God bless you!

Remember , the answer to a linear life is to become creative!

Anissa Sutton

CONTRIBUTORS

FOUNDER
Anissa Sutton

MUSIC REVIEW BY
A. Scott Galloway

FASHION
Tiffani Sutton

MARKETING
Grace Rose
Carter Kaya

PARTNERS

Editions L.A.
www.editions-la.com

The Sound Of L.A.
www.thesoundofla.com

Info Music
www.infomusic.fr

Delit Face
www.DelitFace.com

L.A. Unlimited
www.launlimitedinc.com

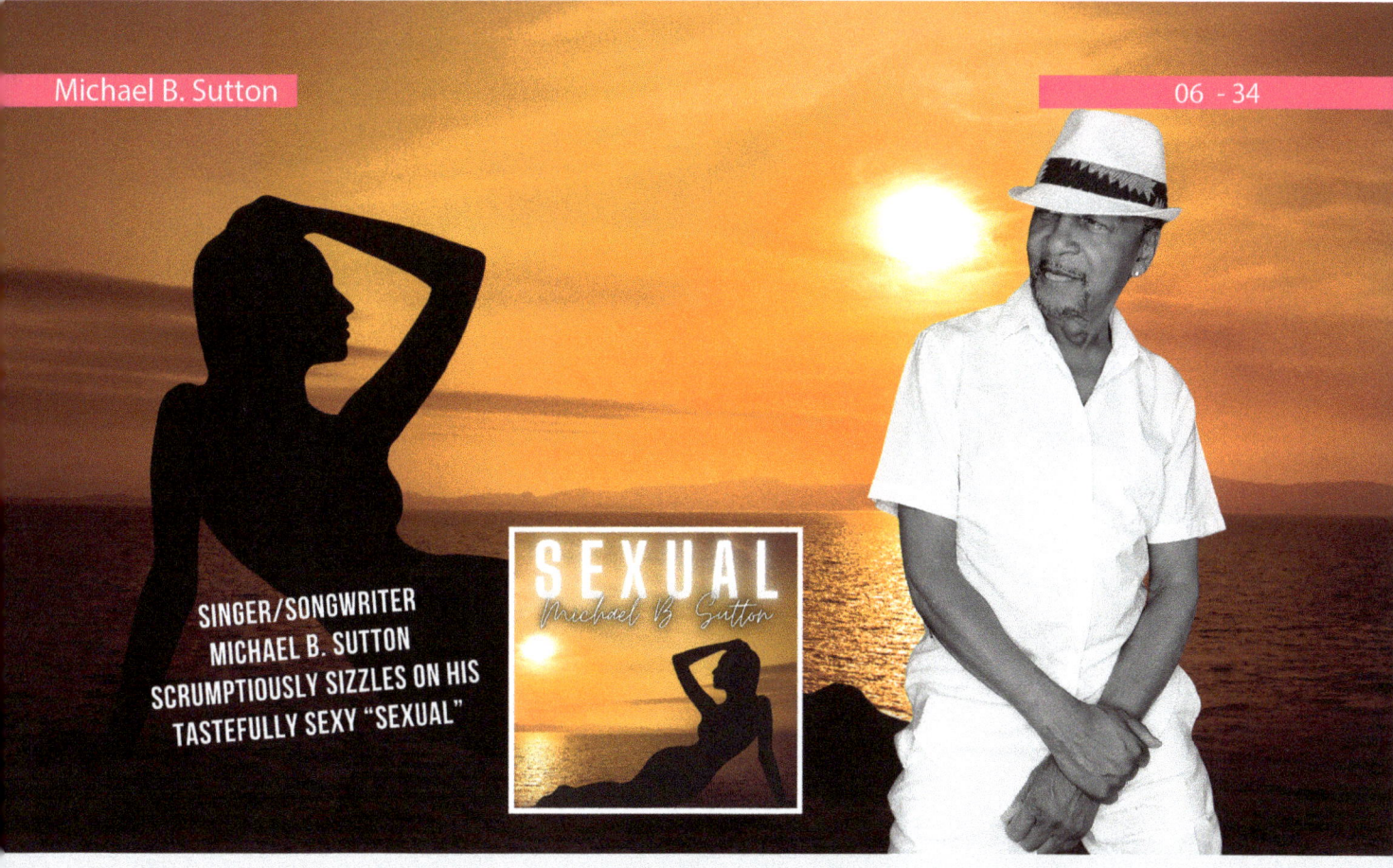

SINGER/SONGWRITER MICHAEL B. SUTTON SCRUMPTIOUSLY SIZZLES ON HIS TASTEFULLY SEXY "SEXUAL"

Singer/Songwriter Michael B. Sutton has mischievously taken some sultry musical steps to ensure that amorous couples can postpone using electric blankets this Fall with his sho' `nuff soulful grown folks' groove, "Sexual."
Lyrically, this most righteous jam is the more up-tempo answer record to Marvin Gaye's 5 A.M. morning lovin' classic "Sexual Healing," playing like a latter-days Johnnie Taylor on Malaco Records sock-feet house par-tay kind of groove! Musically, most people will liken the song to a modern spin on James Brown, The J.B.'s and Horny Horns maestro Fred Wesley's 1973 Funk nugget "Doing it to Death (We're Gonna Have a Funky Good Time)!"

Asked precisely what the inspiration for composing the song and the seventy-something singer chuckles while confessing, "Having a young wife! I have always liked that J.B.'s groove so I decided to write something to it that's sexy but not degrading – something natural…magical…electrical! I wrote it some years ago with singer/actress/playwright Wendy Young (daughter of famed "Mr. Ed" TV show actor Alan Young). I wanted to cut a set of steamy songs for my second CD so we wrote some including that one. However, I never completed the album, so the song went on the shelf. I started thinking about 'Sexual' again recently - for the reason I described above – so now I've finally recorded it…purposefully."

More than a singer, Sutton is a hitmaking songwriter/producer who has written songs for Michael Jackson, Diana Ross and many more. He put all of his precious skills and some new ones to work at the service of "Sexual," including handling the engineering mix himself. Michael is joined on the song by his lovely wife, Anissa who sings background vocals, Josh Sklair on guitar, James Manning on bass, Timbale Cornwell on percussion and Hiroshi Upshur on keys who also arranged the humorously cheesy 'vintage' synthesized horns and strings. Sutton also plays keyboards on the track which was mastered by James Forbes.

"Sexual" is the latest in a teasing string of singles leading to the two-decades-awaited release of Michael B. Sutton's as-yet-untitled second album (his first since 2002's Hopeless Romantic on which Wendy Young also co-wrote "Love Me Inside Out"). No doubt Indian Summer shall continue…between the sheets!
Website: www.thesoundofla.com

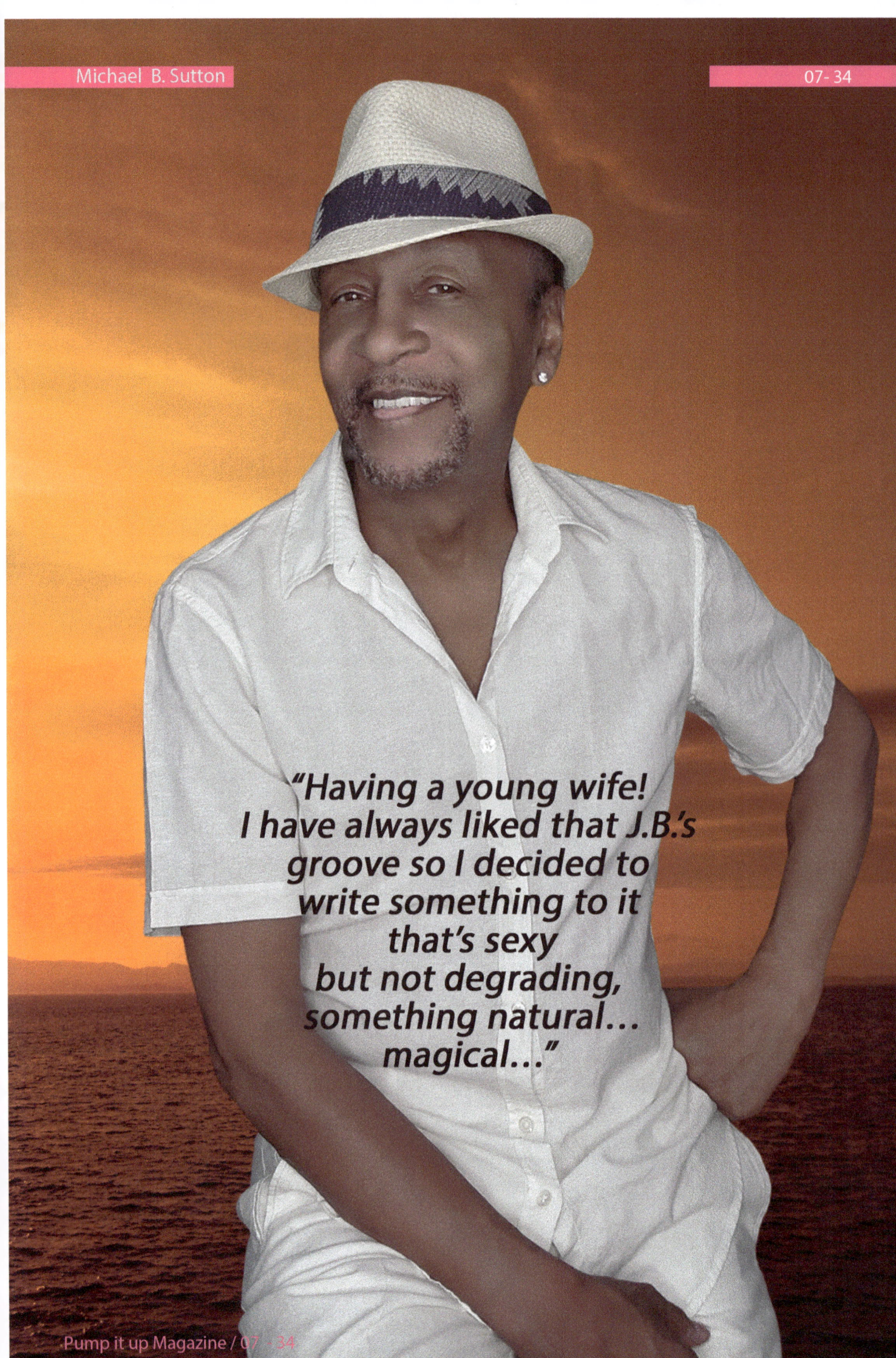

ANEESSA
MICHAEL B. SUTTON

I FOUND MYSELF IN YOU
COMING SOON
SUBSCRIBE NOW

WWW.THESOUNDOFLA.COM

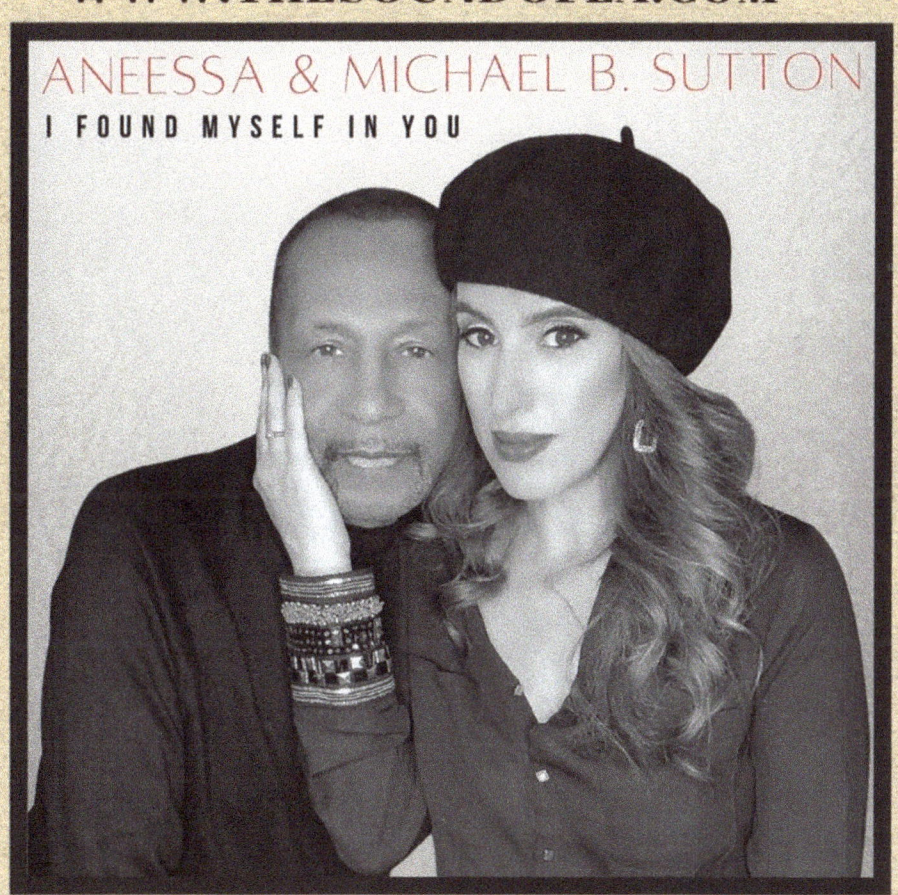

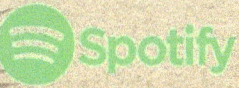   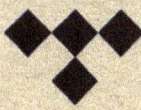 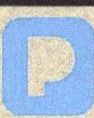 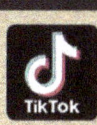

*Smooth Jazz Love Song
for An Essential Romantic Playlist
Capturing the joyful essence of
what it feels like
to love and be loved!*

Sticks & Stones" turns the age-old adage on it's head by adding a funkadelic vibe to it, bringing a positive energy that is very much needed in the world right now!

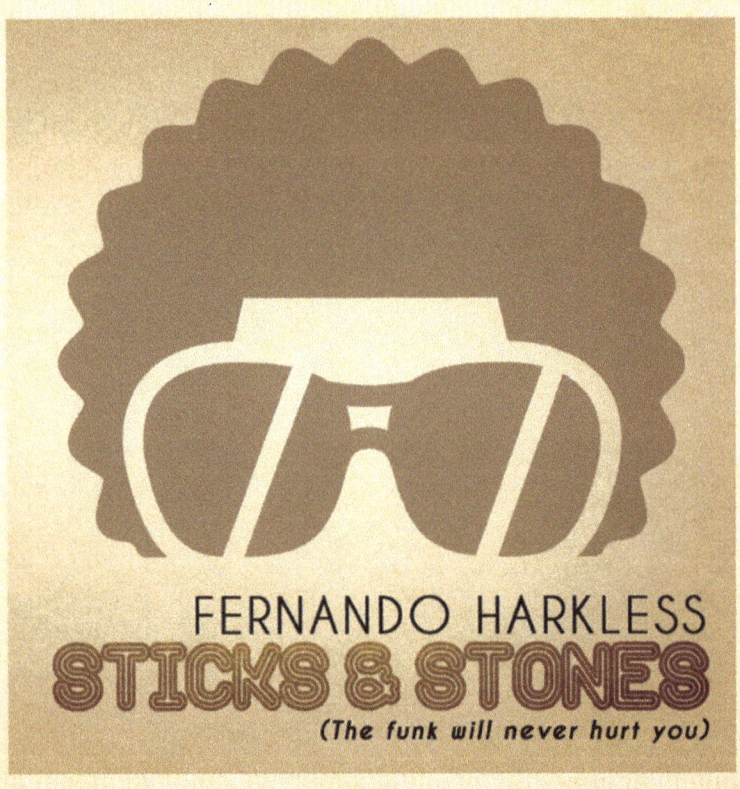

IN STORES NOW

@thesoundofla
WWW.THESOUNDOFLA.COM

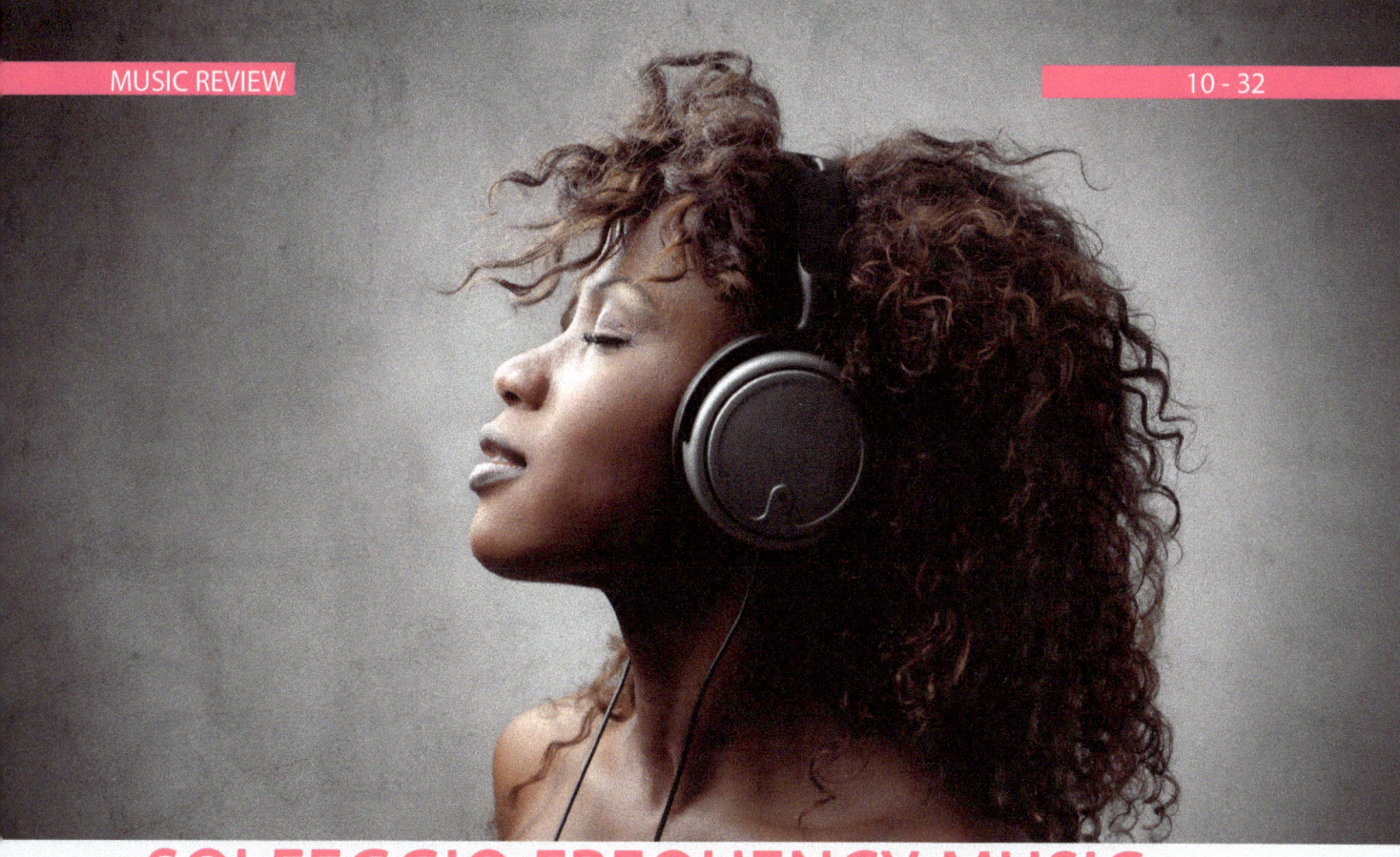

SOLFEGGIO FREQUENCY MUSIC A NATURAL PAINKILLER?

Every sound and every vibration has its own energy and own effect on the body and mind of living beings. The frequency of every sound works differently on the human body and now a recent study has proved that particular frequency music can heal many kinds of diseases and health-related issues.

This article is dedicated to healing music and Solfeggio music that how 174 Hz Solfeggio Frequency music can help relieve pain. Solfeggio music is often used for relieving pain, enhancing meditation's concentration, relieving stress, mind exercise and for yoga practice. That's why it is being called healing music as well.
Our nature has its own harmony and waves, which is roaming around the whole atmosphere. The human body is like an empty vessel and whenever it comes to get contact with these waves and energy, it has amazing effects on the body as well as mental status. Listening to a special kind of music on a special kind of frequency works as an anesthetic and a healer component which helps to generate the awakening mode and one can cure body pain easily and quickly.

Solfeggio music is one of the effective ways to reduce pain and develop a huge sense of love and courage inside you. 174 Hz Solfeggio music directly works on the chakras. Different chakras have different quality and according to spirituality human body contains 7 chakras. One can't be able to see these chakras directly but can be able to awake these chakras with deep Meditation and Pranayama. A person with an enlightened chakras is called an enlightened person which is quite rare.
Healing with sound and music is not a new phenomenon. From ancient time people used to listen to music for relaxation and better sleep.

Based on over 45 years of study and research on millions of people, the solfeggio frequency music is recognized for curing migraine, back pain, legs, and knee pain, enhancing courage and energy of the inner body. Let's take a closer look at some other benefits of solfeggio frequency music:

174 Hz Solfeggio frequency music is highly beneficial and effective for relieving pain. It appears as a natural anesthetic and helps to cure your sick aura around you.

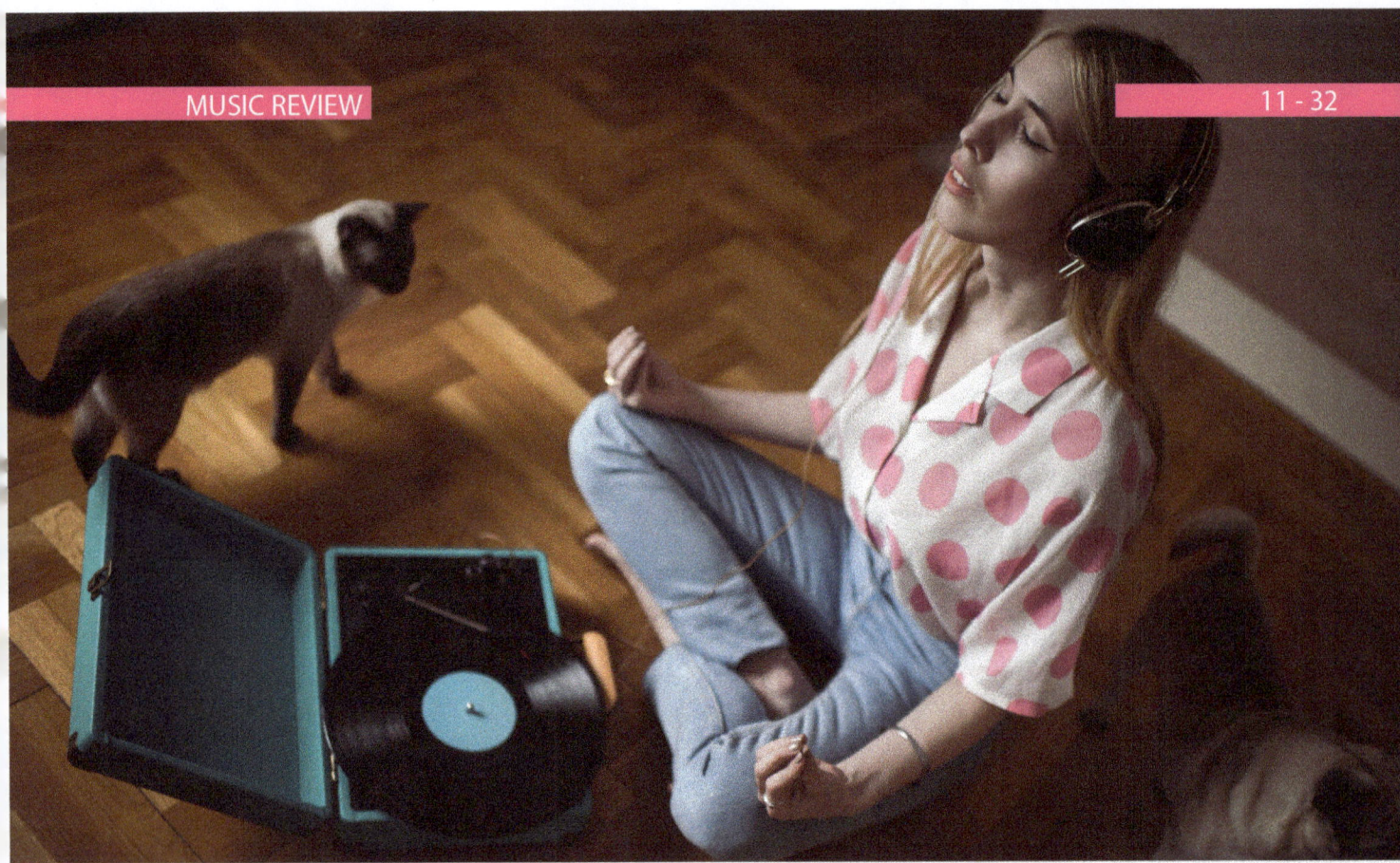

BENEFITS OF SOLFEGGIO FREQUENCY MUSIC

74 Hz Solfeggio frequency music help to relieve back pain, foot pain, leg pain, lower back pain and migraine and stress.
It works like magic on your brain tissues and enhances the emotional power which encourages the sense of safety, love, and courage and helps to cure a person quickly.
174 Hz solfeggio music is the finest source for better concentration level.
174 Hz frequency music contains different nodes and background tones which directly affects the chakras and develops the healing power and energy that makes you feel better.
174 Hz solfeggio frequency music is an excellent way to reduce emotional pain as well. The people who have lost someone or forgot to live happily can get the positive results with this music mode.

THE HEALING ABILITY OF 174HZ MUSIC

Many skepticals ignore the benefits and effects of solfeggio frequency music.

But a recent study at Harvard University has been proved that the patients listening to the solfeggio frequency music were recovering fast and their mental status was far better than non-listener.

174Hz music especially helps in relieving pain as it works like a natural anesthesia and doctors were amazed to find an important fact during surgery that those patients who were listening to healing music during surgery needed less anesthetic dose and they felt less pain during and after surgery.

Listen to OM Mantra Chants at a very low 174 Hz frequency.

OM – The Sound That Reverberates across the universe. The Sound which brings beauty to every cell of our body.

AUM or OM, no matter how you write it, its the inner sound of cosmos. And we have combined it with powerful Solfeggio frequency which is known for its benefits in Pain Relief.

YOUR MUSIC CONSULTANT

"YOU BELIEVE, SO DO WE!"

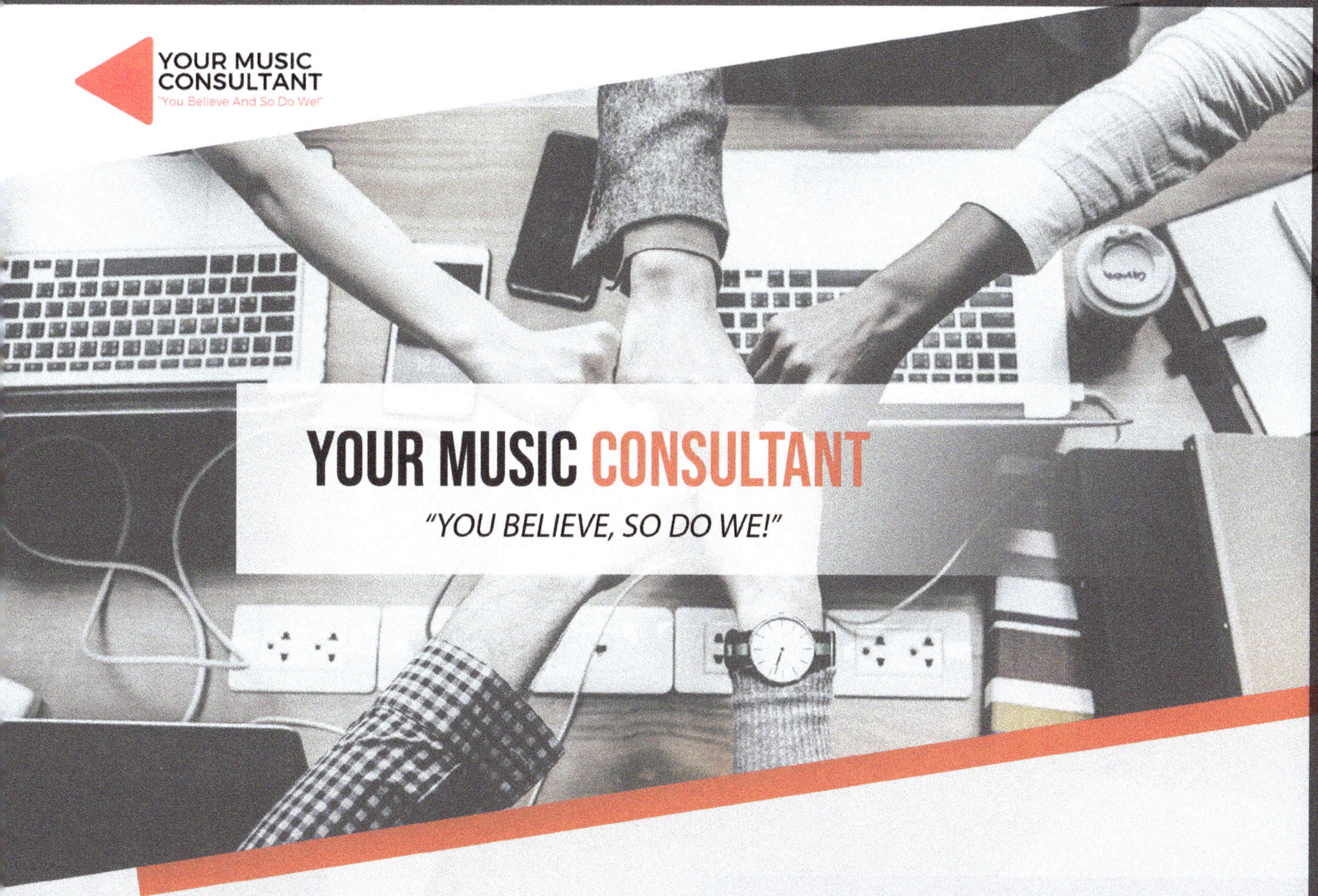

We Can Help You To Grow Your Business

We are a monthly based service, we put faith in artists who has major potential, believed in them, and who are willing to spend their time and own money to work with us in building a successful music career!

Why Choose Us ?

3 DECADES OF MUSIC BUSINESS EXPERIENCE
Platinum and Gold Records
MOTOWN RECORDS
UNIVERSAL
SONY
CAPITOL RECORDS

WE WORKED WITH:
Kanye West - Jay Z - Stevie Wonder - Michael Jackson - Germaine Jackson - Smokey Robinson - Dionne Warwick - Cheryl Lynn - The Originals -

Digital Marketing Services

SOCIAL MEDIA - STREAMING SERVICES - MUSIC DISTRIBUTION - PRESS RELEASE - PRESS DISTRIBUTION - PR

Radio Airplay and TV Commercial

TERRESTRIAL AND DIGITAL RADIO CAMPAIGN AL GENRES EXCEPT HEAVY METAL -
CABLE TV AND MAJOR NETWORK COMMERCIAL

Licensing & Booking

CONCERTS, LIVE MUSIC, EVENTS, CLUB NIGHTS - RED CARPETS -
FOREIGN LICENSING AND SUBOPUBLISHING

📞 **1-818-514-0038**
(Ext. 1)
Monday - Friday / 9am to 6pm

FIND US :

www.YourMusicConsultant.com
30721 Russell Ranch Road Suite 140 Westlake Village, USA
Email : info@yourmusicconsultant.com

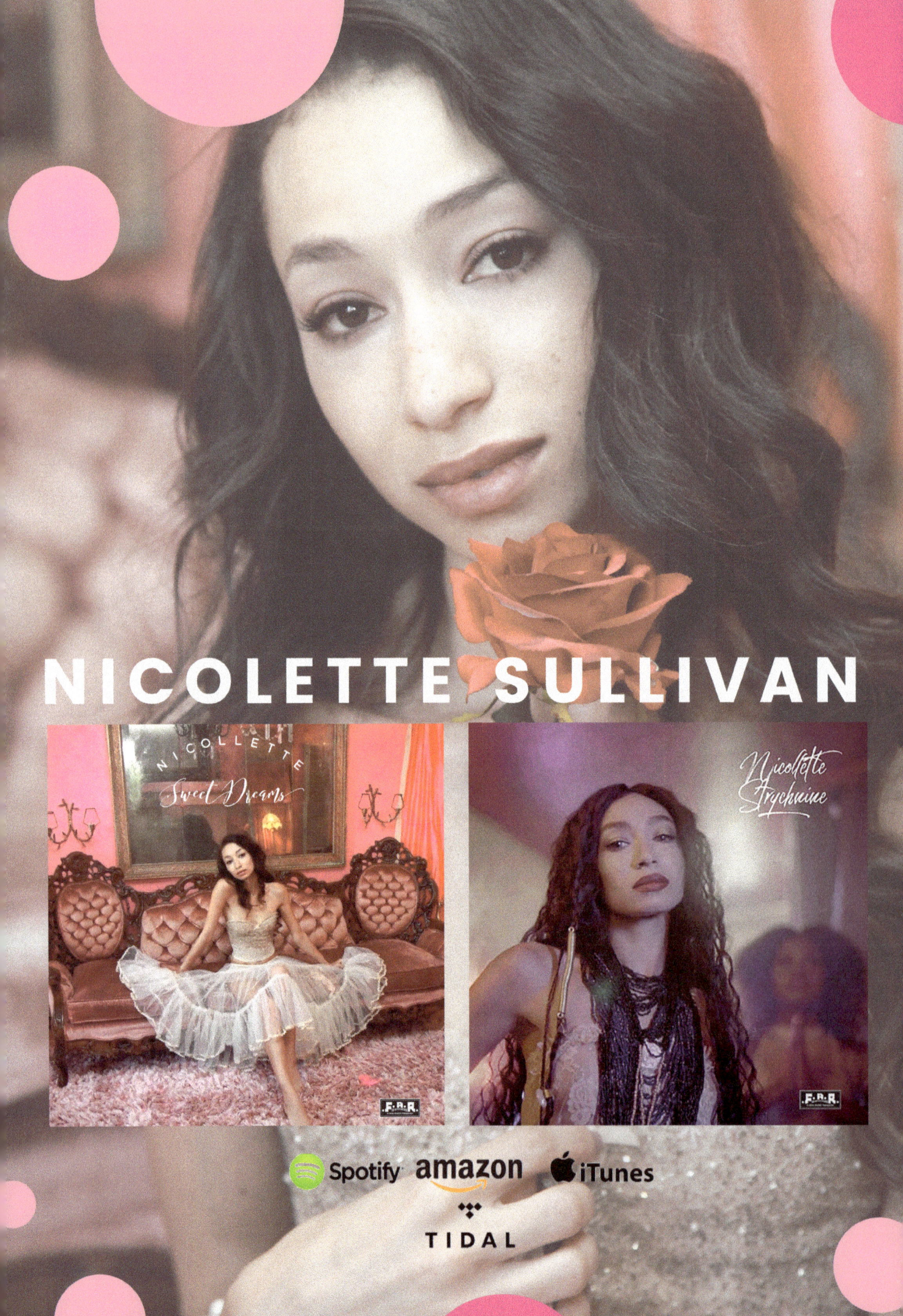

Sexy Loved Filled Bluesy/R&B Song

MICHAEL B. SUTTON

"Feelin' Down"
(Go Down on Me Blues)

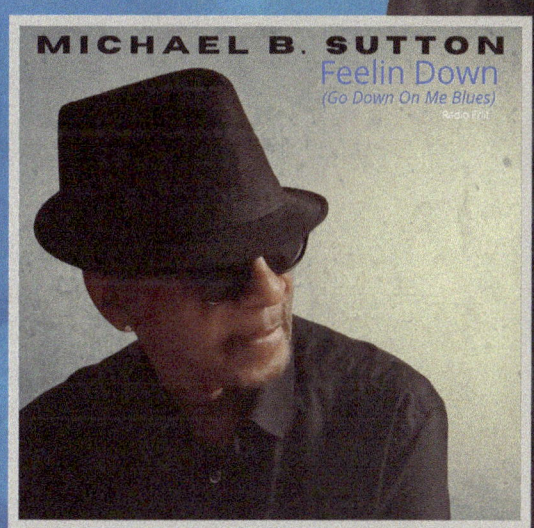

SOUL - R&B - BLUES

MICHAEL B. SUTTON
FEELIN' DOWN (GO DOWN ON ME BLUES)

As a musical veteran, former motwon producer Michael B. Sutton demonstrates his timelessness as an artist in this superb offering Feelin Down (Go Down On Me Blues).
OFFICIAL WEBSITE: WWW.THESOUNDOFLA.COM
FOLLOW MICHAEL B. SUTTON ON SOCIAL MEDIA @MICHAELBSUTTON

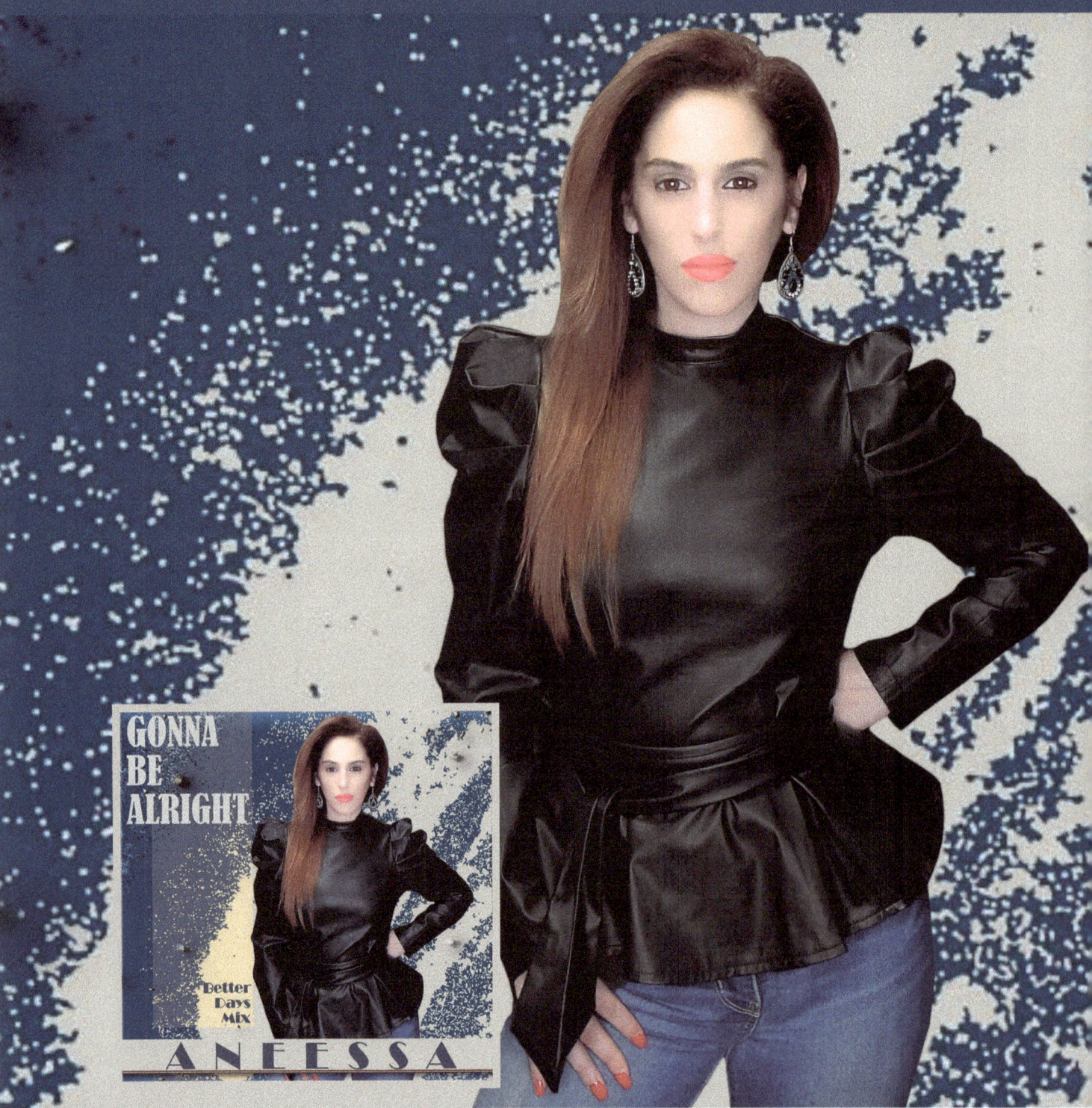

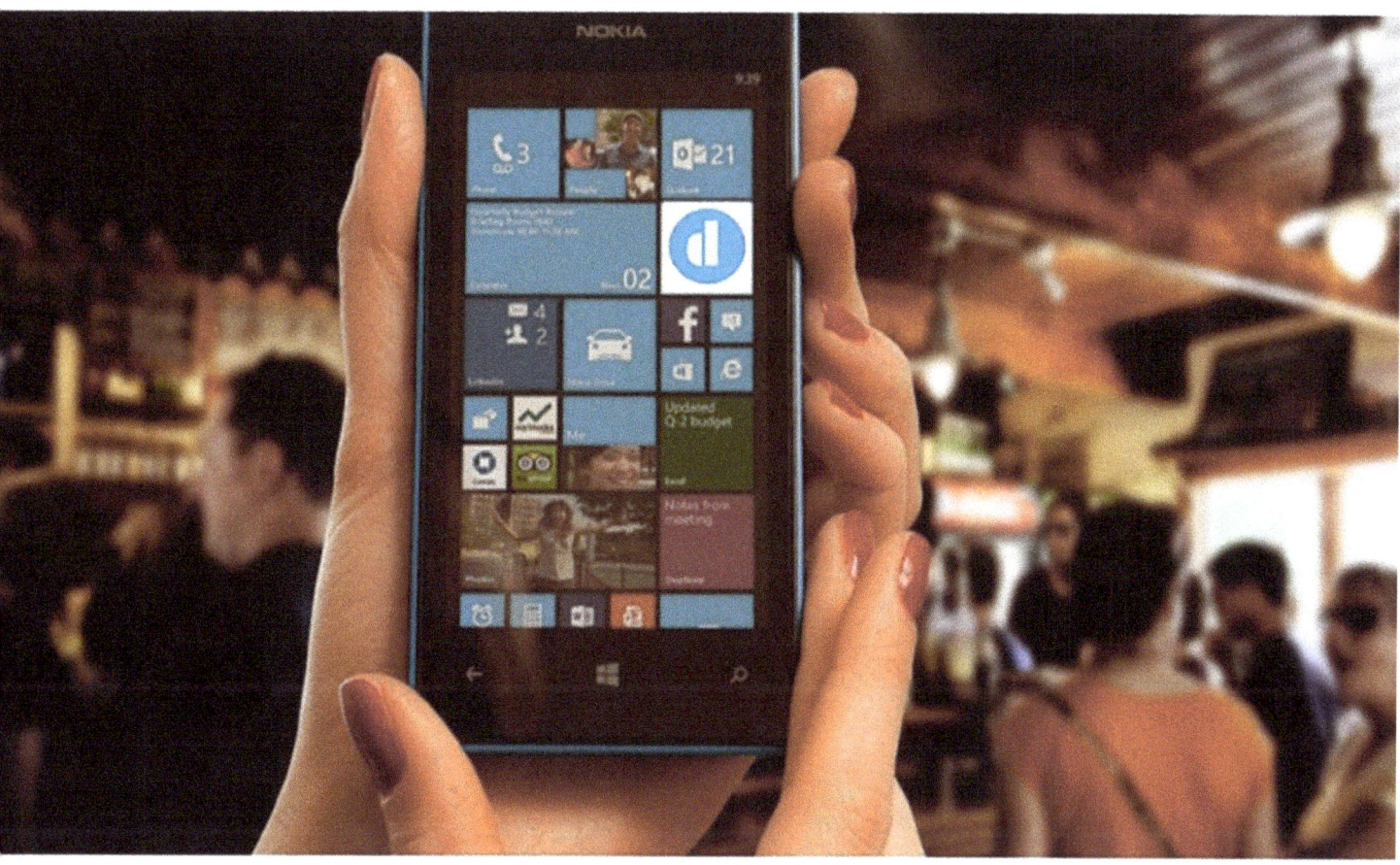

TOP Pump it up

TOP INDIE ARTISTS

R&B - POP - SOUL - BLUES MUSIC

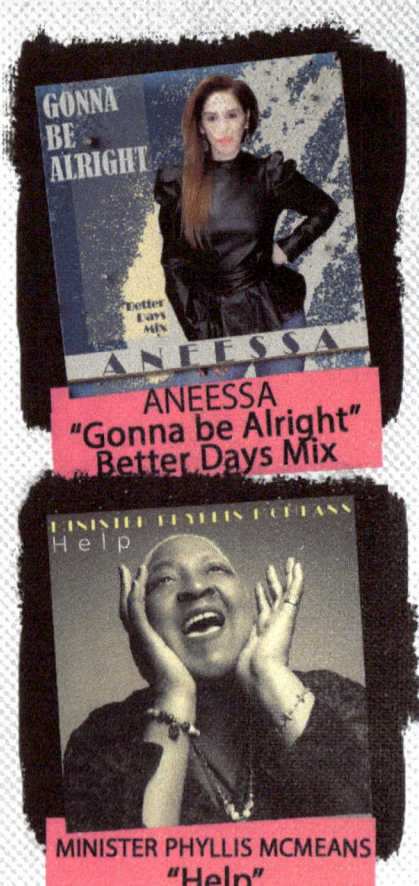

ANEESSA
"Gonna be Alright"
Better Days Mix

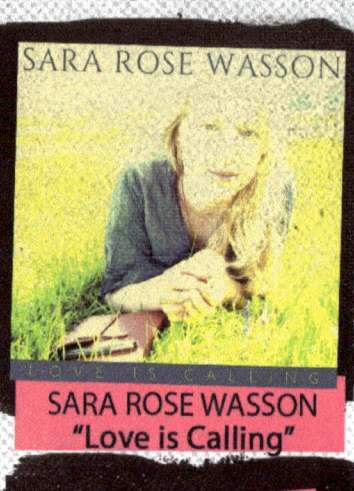

SARA ROSE WASSON
"Love is Calling"

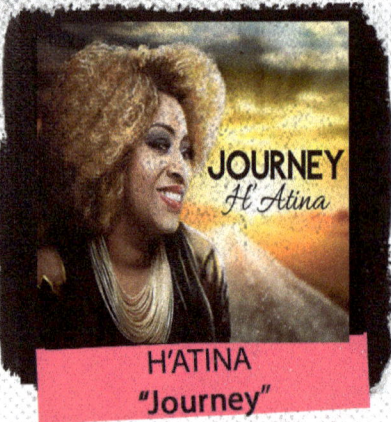

H'ATINA
"Journey"

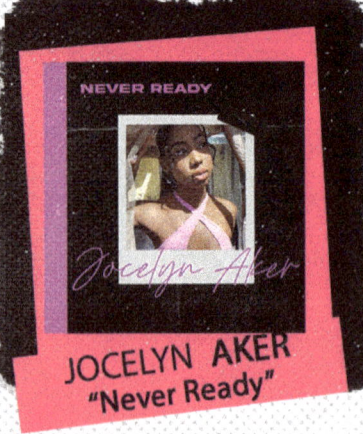

MINISTER PHYLLIS MCMEANS
"Help"

JOCELYN AKER
"Never Ready"

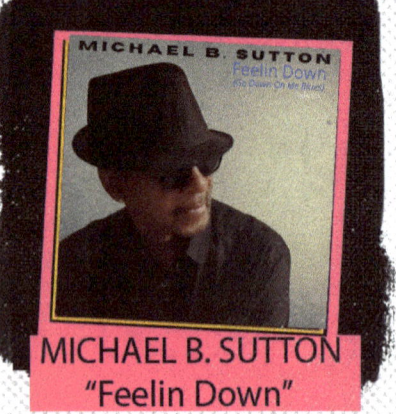

MICHAEL B. SUTTON
"Feelin Down"

TUNE IN ON
PUMP IT UP MAGAZINE RADIO

👍 Pumpitupmag   📷 Pumpitupmagazine   # Pumpitupmagazine.

WWW.PUMPITUPMAGAZINE.COM

Enjoy The Sound Of
Pump it up
RADIO

Get the free Pump it up magazine Radio App on your smartphone or tablet, and you'll never miss your favourite music !

POP - ROCK - DANCE - RNB - JAZZ
Available on Google Play Store

www.PumpItUpMagazine.com

DIGITAL RADIO TRACKER

Leading global broadcast monitoring source that tracks radio airplay of songs in the US and worldwide on more than 5000+ radio stations.

Register for a FREE DRT Account Now!

DIGITALRADIOTRACKER.COM
INFO@DIGITALRADIOTRACKER.COM

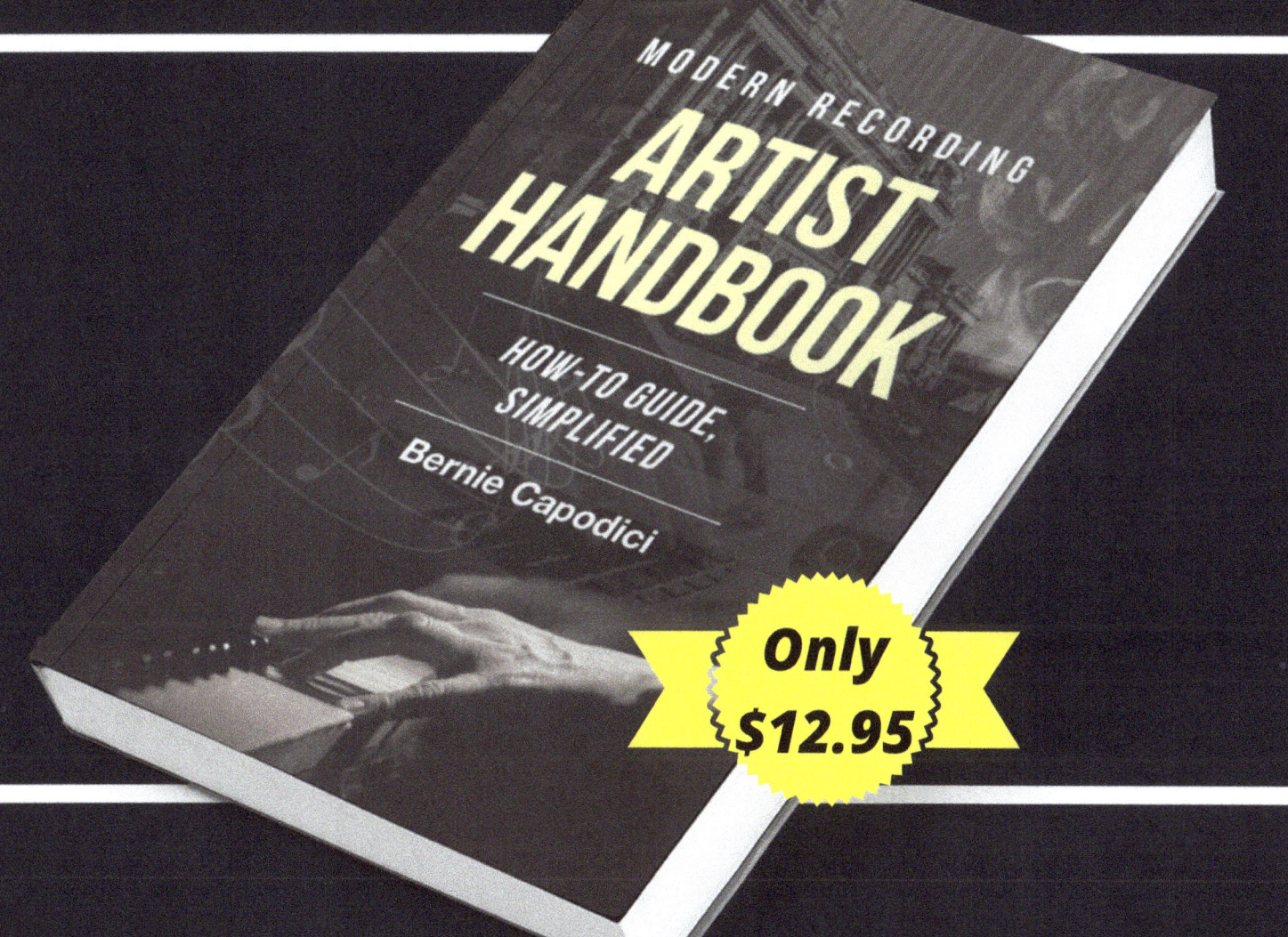

L.A. UNLIMITED

APPAREL REPRESENTATION WITHOUT LIMITS...

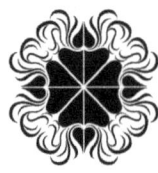

- Corporate Brand Representation
- Brand Identity & Management
- Brand Consulting
- Trade Show Preparation & Participation
- Trunk Shows
- Private Label Sales
- Production Sourcing

L.A. Unlimited & Associates
30765 Pacific Coast Hwy STE 443Malibu, CA 90265

310.882.6432
sales@launlimitedinc.com

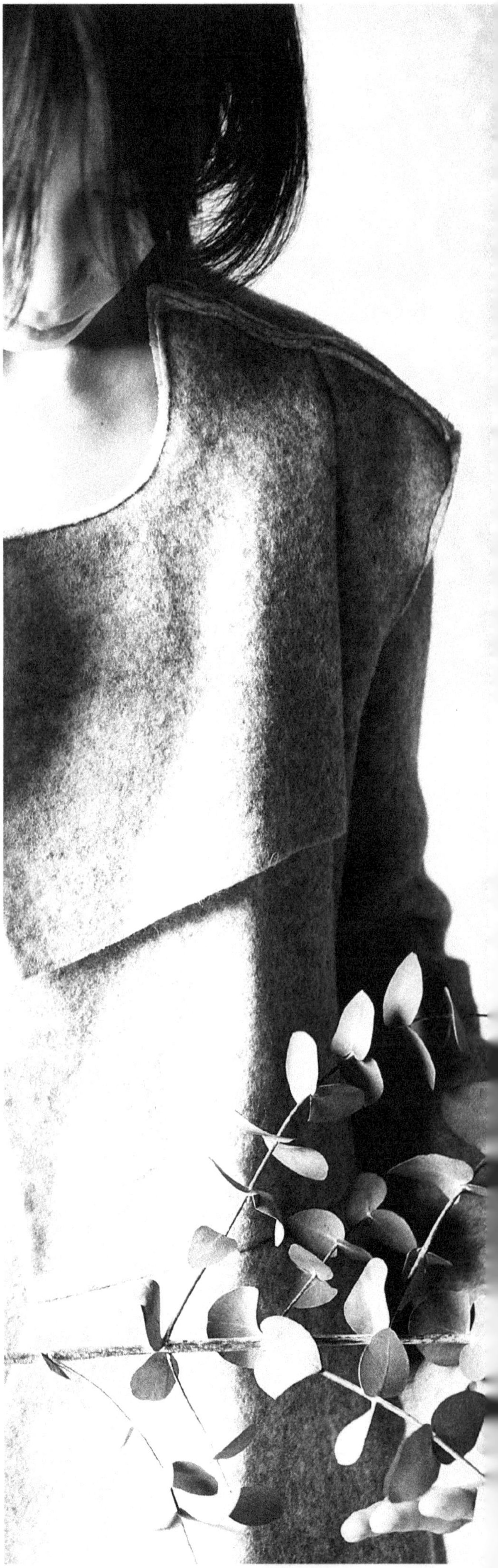

Funk Therapy

| Funky | Trendy | Cool | Hip |

Wear The Music You Love!

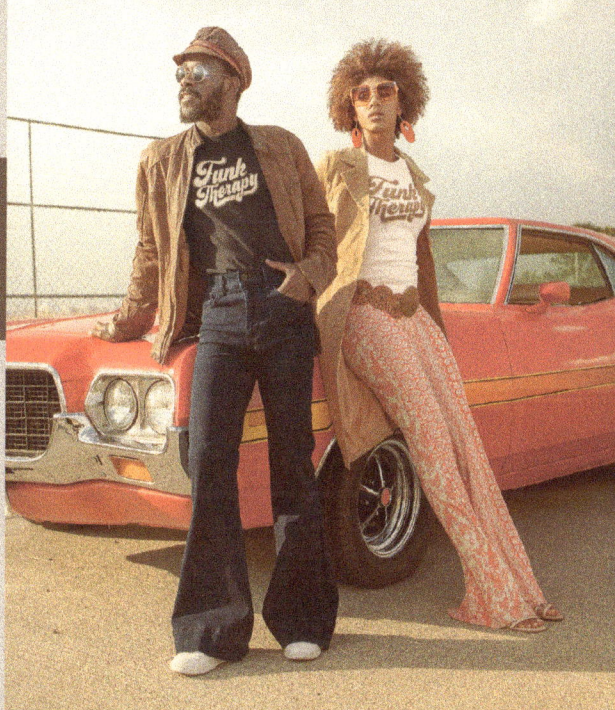

Visit our merchandise store on our website:

WWW.FUNKTHERAPYMUSIC.COM

10% Discount code: STAYFUNKY

- Hoodies
- Crop Top
- Sweat Pants
- Bucket Hats
- Slides
- Mugs

UNISEX T-SHIRTS

Brown T-Shirt
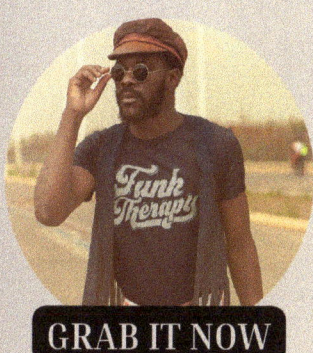
GRAB IT NOW

Orange T-Shirt
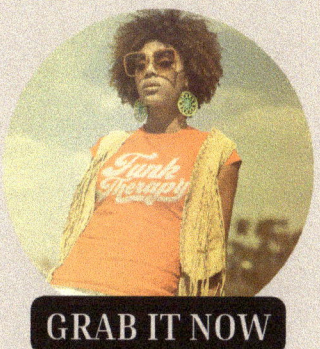
GRAB IT NOW

Beige T-Shirts
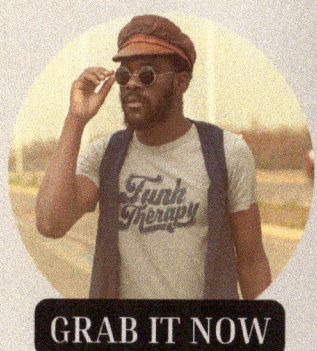
GRAB IT NOW

Join our community
@funktherapy2

FASHION & BEAUTY

HOW TO LOOK EXPENSIVE ON A BUDGET

1. WEAR BLACK

Black is a neutral, it goes with everything. Since it is a solid color it coordinates with other colors and patterns. When we think of the color black, we think of Coco Chanel. She made the colors black and white famous in her tailored clothes and fabrics.

2. MONOCHROME IT OUT

One of the easiest ways to add extra spice to an outfit is with tonal or monochrome pieces. Theodora often styles her clients in identical colored tops and skirts while changing the textures to add a bit of dimension. Monochrome outfits are not only incredibly elongating, but they look effortless, put together, and very expensive.

3. ADD A BLAZER

Amanda Greyson, style director at Free People, believes blazers are the surefire way at elevating even the simplest of outfits. "Try adding a blazer to a simple hoodie and denim look, finishing with a baseball hat and high-top trainers," she suggests. "This will instantly make your look feel more luxe for all those weekend errands. Or, for date night, add an oversized blazer to a silk black dress and easy bootie."

4. WEAR PIECES THAT FIT WELL

Always make sure your clothes fit well. If you have an hourglass figure, wear pieces that fit showing off your curves. If you have a few pounds in areas you want to conceal, opt for pieces that are slightly loose and flow when you walk. For all figures, avoid wearing clothes that are too loose..

5. SPLURGE ON A STRONG BLACK COAT

Invest in classic, high-quality outerwear in timeless black or camel colorways. It will last you decades. Classic styles never expire and will carry you through every decade—warm.

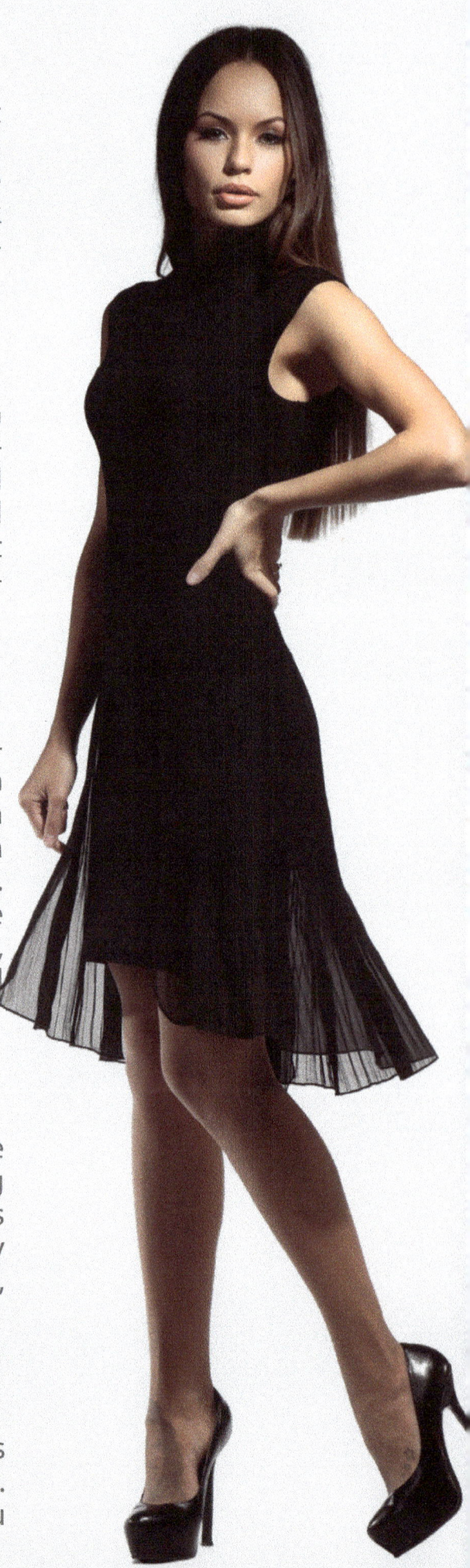

FASHION & BEAUTY

6. WEAR POINTED FLATS OR HEELS

Women who wear flats or heels that are pointed have a look that screams expensive! Black or nude are popular colors that go with everything. They are considered wardrobe essentials.

6. WEAR LIPCOLOR

Wear makeup that looks natural and wear lipcolor. Wear a lipcolor that has a colored tint, like red, coral or pink. Red is a classic lipcolor. It goes great with black and white. Wear a shade of red that looks good with your skin tone. Make sure your nails are kept trimmed and/or painted.

7. COORDINATE YOUR SHOES & BAG

A key to making your outfits look polished is coordinating your shoes and bag. If you wear black shoes then carry a black bag. Brown shoes look great with a brown bag in the same color tone. You can venture out a bit by wearing black shoes with a nude or a solid color bag, like pink. Leopard flats or heels look great with a black or nude bag.

8. WEAR SUNGLASSES

Wear sunglasses and you'll look cool and collected! Perhaps the images of celebrities wearing beautiful sunglasses have been an influence to us to wear them.
The fancier the sunglasses help make your outfit look expensive. black sunglasses, aviator sunglasses, cat-eye sunglasses, leopard sunglasses

9. WEAR STATEMENT JEWELRY

Wear jewelry that makes a statement. Fancy jewelry adds a polished look to any outfit. When your outfit is basic, like black pants and white top, add a statement necklace, earrings bracelet and you outfit instantly looks "glam"!

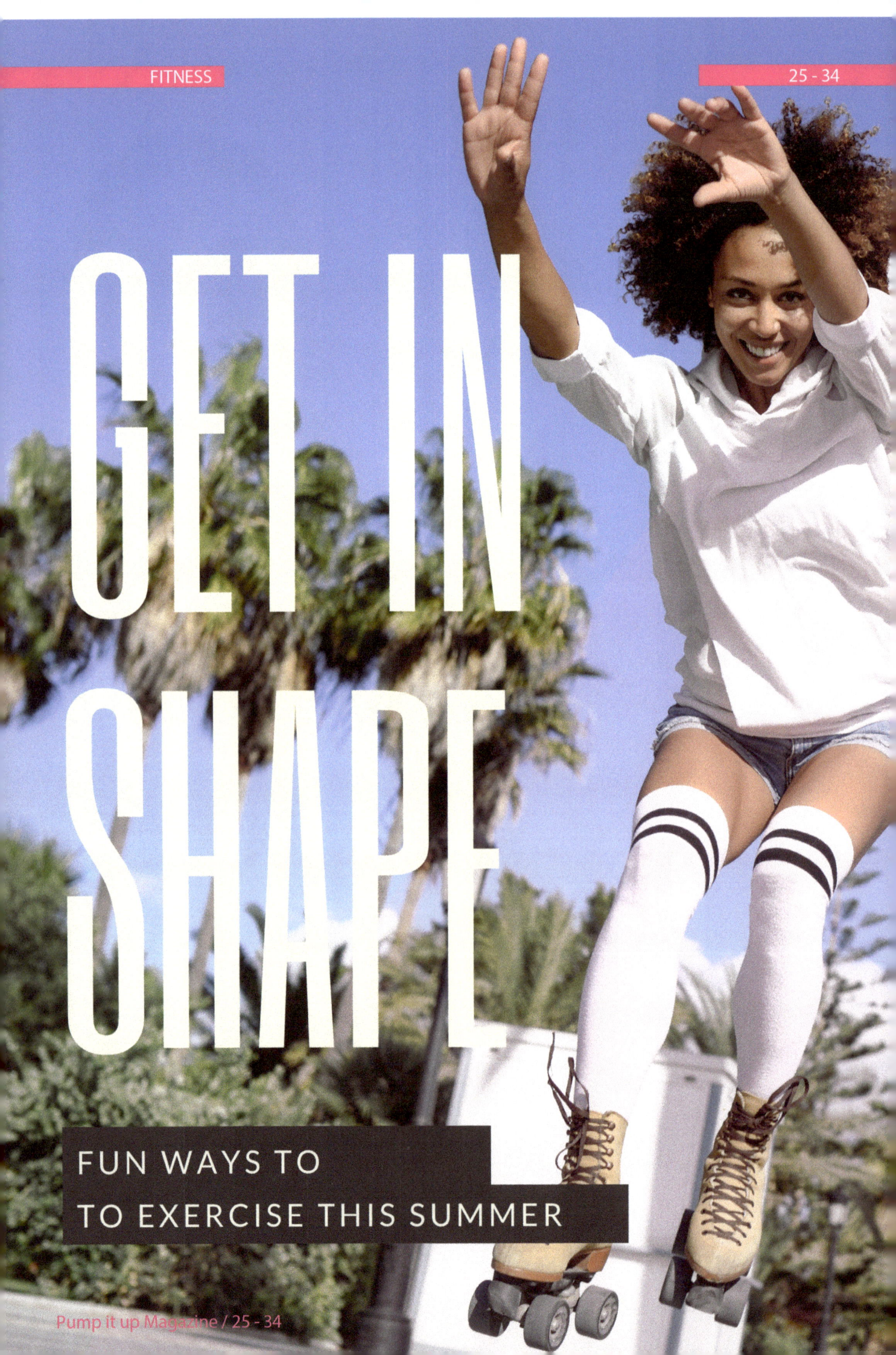

EXERCISE IN SUMMER THAT WON'T FEEL LIKE A CHORE!

ROLLERSKATING — 1
Roller skating is an aerobic workout that increases coordination and balance. This retro pastime doesn't just look cool, it also leaves your body feeling great.

BIKE RIDE — 2
Whether you're one of our crazy intense cyclers in our PK fam, or just down for a slower family ride along the beach- biking is an excellent workout, and so much fun!

FAVORITE CHILDHOOD GAME — 3
Nothing like taking yourself back to days when the living was easy! There is a part of me that will never give up on capture the flag no matter how old. I just wish someone would ask me to play (hint, hint).

DANCING (ZUMBA, SWING..) — 4
Ready to try something new? Join a dance class! When you leave I promise you'll be weating up a storm, and the best part is dancing is so fun!

HAVE A WALKING MEETING — 5
Do you often plan meetings with your coworkers to just sit around and talk? Take that meeting outside and talk as you go for a group walk!

HIKING — 6
There is nothing like a good hike, the burn in your legs, the fresh air, the views. Hiking will never feel like a chore to me, more of a release from everyday life!

ACTIVE VIDEO GAMES — 7
Active video games are truly the best! They're so fun, and you can really work up a sweat quick if you do it right!

HAVE FUN!

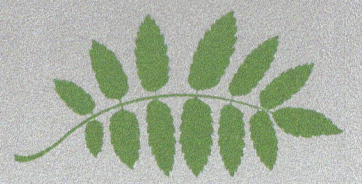

WEST END ORGANIX

Ageless Beauty, Organic Health

Look and feel younger and healthier with our natural remedies products!

www.WestEndOrganix.com

Discount: 10% off of your order - Code *WEO2021*

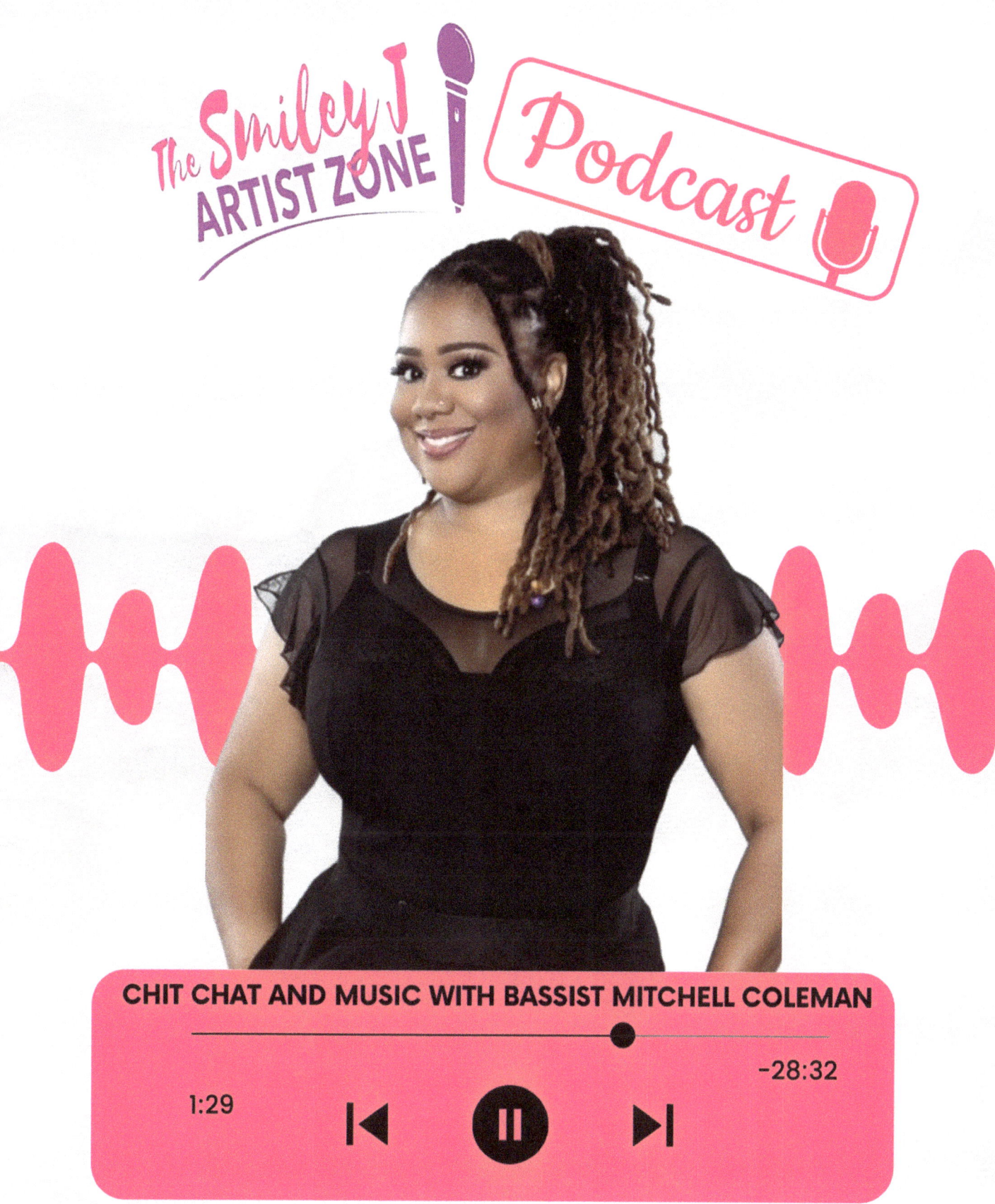

Listen to The Smiley J. Artist Zone
www.thesmileyjartistzone.podbean.com
and on all your favorite streaming platforms!

GAIN CONTROL OF YOUR SUBSCONSCIOUS MIND!

HYPNOTHERAPIST
Nader Hanna

818.445.1646

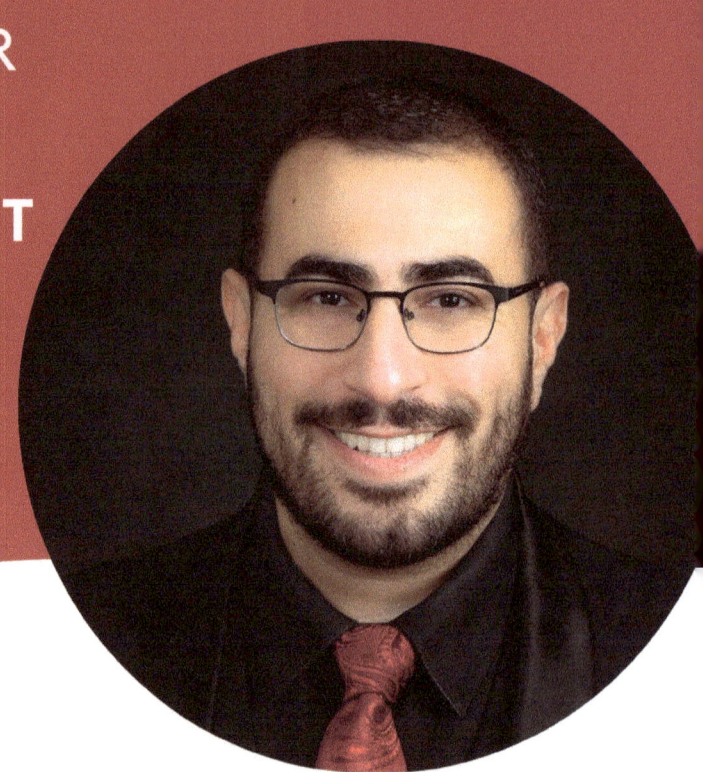

ABOUT

Nader's professionalism, warmth and flexibility coupled with his unique skills make him the perfect hypnotherapist to help you succeed in the positive changes in your life you have been dreaming of!

This Master Hypnotist is known for his mind-bending feats of ESP and hypnosis which he has displayed impressively while performing in shows for big names like John Landis, Joe Dante, Tippi Hedren, and at corporate events for companies such as NBC Universal.

HYPNOSIS WILL HELP YOU WITH

- **FEARS & PHOBIAS**
- **ANXIETY**
- **SPORTS PERFORMANCE**
- **FITNESS**
- **STOP SMOKING**

www.themasterhypnotist.com
www.themastermentalist.com

Los Angeles, California

AWARENESS

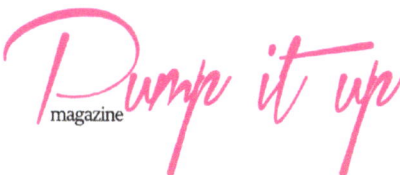

Tips For Taking Care Of Your
MENTAL HEALTH
C-PTSD & NARCISSISTIC ABUSE

People who have Narcissistic Personality Disorder have damaged self-esteem that is easily harmed by even small criticisms.
They are continually looking to shore up their weak areas of self-opinion.
To accomplish this need for self-preservation, they abuse and use other people, including, unfortunately, their own children, significant others etc..

Recognize the trait of the narcissist
A sense of uniqueness
Boastful behavior
Exaggeration of their talents
Grandiose fantasies
A sense of superiority
Self-centered behavior
Self-referential behavior
A deep need for attention and admiration

Recognize the trait of The covert narcissist
Passive Self-Importance
Blaming and Shaming
Creating Confusion
Procrastination and Disregard
(The covert narcissist is a professional at not acknowledging you at all.)
Giving With a Goal (to make themselves look good)
Emotionally Neglectful

How to Deal With a Narcissist
Set Boundaries
Avoid Taking It Personally
Advocate for Yourself
Create a Healthy Distance
Seek Help - Talk to a Therapist
Remove the Heart Wall
Emotion Codean energy healing technique for releasing trapped emotion

C-PTSD
Complex Post Traumatic Stress Disorder
is more severe if:
the traumatic events happened early in life
the trauma was caused by a wife/husband/parent
the person experienced the trauma for a long time
the person was alone during the trauma
there's still contact with the person responsible for the trauma

Symptoms of complex PTSD
Anxiety - Agoraphobia - Panic Attack
Alcoholism - Drug Abuse
Negative thoughts about yourself, other people or the world
Hopelessness about the future
Memory problems,
Difficulty maintaining close relationships
Feeling detached from family and friends
Lack of interest in activities you once enjoyed
Difficulty experiencing positive emotions
Feeling emotionally numb

How to Treat complex PTSD
Set Boundaries
Avoid Taking It Personally
Advocate for Yourself
Create a Healthy Distance
Seek Help - Talk to a Therapist
Remove the Heart Wall
with the help of a Healer

@pumpitupmagazine
www.pumpitupmagazine.com

FUN QUIZZES 31 - 34

MY MUSIC LIST

_____
A SONG THAT MAKES ME HAPPY

_____
A SONG FROM THE 70s

_____
A SONG ABOUT YOUR COUNTRY

_____
A SONG WITH A COLOR

_____
A SONG YOU CAN'T LISTEN ANYMORE

SHARE THIS LIST WITH YOUR FRIENDS

ALBUM CHALLENGE

_____
DEBUT ALBUM

_____
CONCEPT ALBUM

_____
80'S ALBUM

_____
LIVE ALBUM

_____
SOUNDTRACK

_____
FAVORITE ALBUM

This or That

What would you choose?

Get up early or Stay up late

Talk to dogs or Talk to cats

Lose your sense of taste or Lose your sense of smell

Give up on music or Give up on movies

Read minds or Know everything

Travel to the future or Travel to the past

WHAT WOULD YOU PREFER...
RANDOM EDITION

Live in the city or Live in the countryside

Play video games or Play board games

Lose your phone or Lose your wallet

Speak many languages or Speak with animals

Own a private island or Own a private jet

Live without music or Live without TV

EATING WELL FOR MENTAL HEALTH

You've probably heard the phrase "Food is Medicine". This famous phrase comes from Ancient Greek physician Hippocrates, "Let food be thy medicine, and let medicine be thy food" and with so many processed and unhealthy options available, it's never been more important.

We all know proper nutrition is good for our bodies. We know it helps us build muscle, stay fit, maintain healthy skin, and keep our energy stable. But somehow we always treat our minds as if they're separate from our bodies, and our mental health separate from the food we eat.

But more and more, we're discovering the direct relationship between our nutrition and our anxiety, depression, clarity, and happiness. It's even developing into its own field Nutritional Psychology. Why? Because our brains are the center of everything.

Think about it. Your brain is always "on." It takes care of your thoughts and movements, your breathing and heartbeat, your senses — it works hard 24/7, even while you're asleep. This means your brain requires a constant supply of fuel. That "fuel" comes from the foods you eat — and what's in that fuel makes all the difference. Put simply, what you eat directly affects the structure and function of your brain and, ultimately, your mood.

What do you eat for Mental Health?

First of all, know that you can't be perfect every day. Sometimes being a little imperfect and enjoying some foods or drinks that are "not ideal for your mental health" is part of living a healthy balanced life.

At MacroPlate.com, we often emphasize the 80/20 rule. Make sure your healthy life choices fill 80% of your lifestyle, and your "live-a-little" choices satisfy that other 20%.

But in general, a diet full of rich plant-based foods with grains, fruits, and veggies, combined with healthy protein sources, and plenty of good clean fats is the best way to go.

However, some foods stand above and beyond others as being nutritionally dense with micronutrients that really benefit and support a healthy mind and mood.

The Best Foods for Mental Health

Oatmeal

While your body and brain utilize carbohydrates for energy, too often we consume simple carbs, which lead to blood sugar spikes. Foods classified as whole grains contain complex carbohydrates, which leads to glucose being produced more slowly, as a more even and consistent source of energy.

Also, oats help the brain absorb tryptophan, which helps reduce the symptoms of depression and anxiety while boosting brain function.

Salmon

Fish, in general, is a healthy choice, but salmon is at the top of the list. It's a "fatty" fish, containing high amounts of omega-3 fatty acids, which have been linked to a reduction in mental disorders such as depression. Omega-3s have been shown to boost learning and memory as well.

AWARENESS

EATING WELL FOR MENTAL HEALTH

Brocoli Sprouts
Broccoli Sprouts are nature's miracle food. So much so, we've already written a whole blog about them. They're actually one of the healthiest plant compounds on earth, with off-the-chart concentrated levels nutrients that have been proven to provide many nutritional benefits from brain-boosting anti-aging, preventing memory loss, treating depression, and improving the brain function of autism.

Walnuts
When eaten in moderation, most nuts are a good source of heart-healthy monounsaturated fats as well as protein. But walnuts get the edge when it comes to lessening the symptoms of depression because they also are one of the richest plant-based sources of omega-3 fatty acids. "The omega-3s in walnuts support overall brain health," says Robin H-C.

Yogurt
Probiotics are beneficial bacteria that exist naturally in foods like yogurt and kimchi. While we're familiar with how they impact our gut health, there's new evidence that they're also really beneficial for our mental health. Studies suggest that probiotics, as found in yogurt, may reduce the risk of depression by boosting the production of serotonin from an amino acid, tryptophan.

Berries
Berries, specifically blueberries and blackberries are full of antioxidants which are outstanding at mitigating depression. And luckily, the effects are immediate. In recent studies, blueberries improved positive affect – a measure of positive moods such as joy, interest, and alertness – 2-hours after consumption.

Banana
Eating potassium-rich foods such, as pumpkin seeds or bananas, may help reduce symptoms of stress and anxiety. They also help with mood balance and depression. The two key components in bananas are vitamin B-6 and tryptophan. Separately, they work to reduce depressive symptoms, and together, they form a dynamic duo of brain chemistry to send you tons of positive vibes.

Chocolate
No, it's not just because chocolate makes us feel good. Dark chocolate can help reduce anxiety and improve symptoms of clinical depression. People who ate dark chocolate in two 24-hour periods had 70% reduced odds of reporting depressive symptoms than those who did not eat chocolate. Remember that the cacao is the important bit, so avoid really milky chocolates that are mostly cream and sugar.

Apricots
Apricots are rich in magnesium, which acts a natural stress-buster and helps to calm tensed muscles. A deficiency of magnesium is known to cause headaches and leaves you fatigued. Apricots contain Vitamin B that helps to cure nervous system disorders like hyperactivity, memory loss and mental fatigue.

www.ingramcontent.com/pod-product-compliance
Lightning Source LLC
Chambersburg PA
CBHW040949020526

44118CB00044B/2820